Gender Dysphoria

An Essential Guide for Understanding and Dealing with Gender Identity Disorder

by Eleanor Nye

Table of Contents

Introduction

You're probably reading this book because you or someone you know has concerns regarding gender identity. It may be that you're biologically male, yet you don't feel comfortable with your gender and you have this persistent desire to act like a female. It may also be that your child is female but she wants to act like a boy. Or, perhaps your husband has shown an obsession with becoming female, and you don't know how to deal with it. Whatever your case may be, just know that you're not alone. Thousands of people all over the globe are now acknowledging conflicts with how they perceive their gender. The best way to resolve how you feel about your gender is to first understand what's causing you to feel this way, and then get to know what your options are.

The behavior aforementioned is a condition called Gender Identity Disorder. Recently, experts re-named it Gender Dysphoria because they came to realize that the condition is not a mental disorder or a pathologic disease, but it's simply something that people go through because of biological causes.

It's important to learn about and understand the issue of Gender Dysphoria because when the desire to be the opposite gender is not fulfilled or addressed, all sorts of emotional and psychological issues then result, including things like anxiety and depression. This may then lead to bigger problems, such as chronic depression or schizophrenia. As you can see, having these feelings must not be ignored. As a person with Gender Dysphoria, you owe it to yourself to address your feelings head on. And as a friend or loved one of someone with Gender Dysphoria, it's critical that you take time to try and understand what your friend or loved one is really going through on the inside. Not acknowledging it or not understanding how to deal with it can cause humiliation, pain and unhappiness.

In this book, you will come to understand what causes Gender Dysphoria, how to recognize the common symptoms, and how the condition can be identified or diagnosed. You will then learn what different options you have for dealing with the situation, which of course depends on your specific individual scenario, whether you're an adult making a personal decision, or whether you're a parent of a child with Gender Dysphoria and you need help figuring out what course of action should be taken next. You will also be introduced to strategies that you can implement at home as well as potential options for medical intervention if that's the path you decide to take. Furthermore, you will become familiarized with laws protecting transgender rights, which will help protect you or your loved one from unnecessary discrimination. And last but not least, I have included a chapter with 15 important pointers that you can refer to whenever you deem necessary.

NOTE: It's important to add that this book was not written to judge you or to persuade you to take one path versus another. It's simply designed to help you better understand what Gender Dysphoria is, and to become more informed about what options you have.

Chapter 1: Causes, Symptoms, and Diagnosis of Gender Dysphoria

The specific cause of Gender (female or male) Dysphoria (feeling of discomfort or discontent) has not yet been specifically established. Previously, it was thought to be a mental disorder; but through the years, experts have found out that it may be more of a biological condition. Though, further studies have to be conducted to identify the specific causes, the following are observed to be associated with Gender Dysphoria.

Causes of Gender Dysphoria

1. Inadequate biological development of fetus

The development of the child's gender starts in the womb when the chromosomes from both parents are inherited by the child. The child inherits 50% of the father's chromosomes and 50% of the mother's. If the father's chromosome is an X chromosome, the child will be female, but if the father's chromosome is a Y chromosome, the child will be male.

As the fetus grows in the womb of the mother, the hormones responsible for the secondary sexual characteristics of the child are increasingly secreted. This is then interpreted by the brain, which reacts accordingly. The brain operates by the stimuli sent from different parts of the body, and a hormonal imbalance will be recognized by the brain, heightening Gender Dysphoria.

For males, the hormones testosterone and androgens produced by the testes and the adrenal cortex are increasingly secreted so that male sexual characteristics are developed, such as proper penis and scrotum growth.

In females, there is an increase in the secretion of estrogen and progesterone to help develop the secondary sexual characteristics, such as the vagina and other female organs. Insufficient amount of these hormones can lead to Gender Dysphoria.

2. Congenital adrenal hyperplasia

The baby may have both the female and male genitalia upon birth, and there will be confusion to what gender he/she belongs too. In this case, the parents will have to decide the baby's gender. This rare condition denotes that the adrenal glands responsible for secreting some of the androgens, which are hormones responsible for a baby's male gender, are hyperactive.

Consequently, intersex conditions or hermaphroditism can also result as an effect of hormonal problems.

In a nutshell, Gender Dysphoria has a biologic cause; hence it's different from homosexuality. The biologic component is the primary factor, while the environment and social interaction the child experiences come as secondary factors.

The symptoms of Gender Dysphoria can vary for each individual, but most commonly observed are these.

Symptoms of Gender Dysphoria

1. Discomfort with one's gender

There's a feeling of discomfort in performing the roles identified with the assigned or birth gender. If the person is male, he attempts to become female by engaging in female activities. If she's female, she's not comfortable fulfilling her role but engages in male events, such as weight lifting, and other manly sports. There's a cross gender identification that affects all aspects of the individual's life.

2. Anxiety

Anxiety results when the person is not allowed to perform their desired activities. The person is anxious up to a point that he (in the case of a male) no longer can concentrate on his obligations at work and at home. If the person is a child, he may throw tantrums and grow anxious every time someone tells him to do something against his perceived gender, which is female.

3. Depression

The person also feels depressed. The only thing that can lift the person up is when he/she participates in activities that enhance his/her preferred gender (not the birth gender).

4. Persistent verbal expression of sex change

He/She expresses verbally his/her desire to be the other gender. This can go on for months. If it's not Gender Dysphoria, the desire will dwindle and vanish; but if it is

11

Gender Dysphoria, the desire persists. Experts observed that a person who usually expresses his/her desire of swapping his/her gender for a minimum of 6 months or more has Gender Dysphoria.

5. Feeling of guilt

There are instances in which individuals with Gender Dysphoria have stopped expressing their desire to be the opposite gender and tend to get married and have children. In these instances, the feeling of guilt becomes intense. If there are no people around them who they can confide in and ask advice from, they may tend to resort to drastic actions. Therefore, it is crucial that these persons have supportive people around them.

Getting married won't eliminate the problem of Gender Dysphoria. It will only exacerbate it because the person will soon realize that the desire is still there. The feeling of having lied to the family will increase as the person stays longer in the marriage. If the person has no will or determination to perform a sex change, then the person may become severely depressed and anxious.

6. Wearing clothes and paraphernalia of the other sex

This is more prevalent in children. They wear the clothes of the opposite sex whenever they have the chance.

7. Participation in events of the other sex

During games and events, the individuals participate in the other sex's games, and also prefer to play with the gender they want to be. If he were a boy, he would want to play with girls, and would prefer dolls and other girly activities.

8. Persistent preference of the secondary sexual characteristics of the other gender

If the person is female, she may want to acquire a deep voice, facial hair, an Adam's apple, a penis, a scrotum, and the muscular build of a male. If the person is male, he may want to develop breasts, possess a vagina, a feminine voice and other feminine traits.

13

9. Rejection and feeling of disgust over one's assigned gender

The person doesn't acknowledge his penis or her vagina but despises it. Likewise, he/she will insist that his/her organ is of the other sex. The individual feels disgusted by his/her own organ and tries to hide it through the style of clothing.

The feelings involved are typically dominant and persistent. If these are transitory, then it may not be Gender Dysphoria.

If you want to confirm your suspicions, you should consult with a competent health professional, who has had experience with this condition. An accurate diagnosis can only happen if the person suffering from Gender Dysphoria is honest about how he/she really feels.

Diagnosis of Gender Dysphoria

Diagnosis of the condition can be done through analyzing the following:

1. Personal history

The health professional or medical doctor will conduct an assessment of the person's personal history, his/her symptoms and other underlying factors. This is a vital factor in the correct diagnosis of Gender Dysphoria because the symptoms are commonly evaluated through the personal history of the individual. When there are 3 or more symptoms demonstrated by the person, then he/she is diagnosed with Gender Dysphoria.

2. Medical history

The doctor will evaluate the medical history of the patient and may request diagnostic laboratory tests to determine whether there are some diseases that may have caused the condition. A laboratory test for male and female hormones, such as testosterone and androgens for males, and estrogen and progesterone for females can help with the diagnosis. Any increase or decrease of these hormones can confirm or reject the initial diagnosis of Gender Dysphoria.

These are important information that you must know about Gender Dysphoria. They will help you understand more about what the condition is all about.

Chapter 2: Dealing with Gender Dysphoria

Dealing with Gender Dysphoria will vary depending on the choices of the individuals. If they are adults, they should decide what they want to do next. If the person is still a minor, the parents should decide what's best for their child. The following are recommended steps in dealing with Gender Dysphoria.

Step #1 – Obtain a definite diagnosis from a team of health specialists

Seek expert opinion first before proceeding with any plans that you have. The condition has to be confirmed as Gender Dysphoria by competent specialists from various disciplines, who are experts on the condition. You can consult with a multi-disciplinary team (MDT), which are commonly composed of a medical doctor, a psychoanalyst, psychologist and a psychiatrist for accurate diagnosis. Once the diagnosis is confirmed, you can proceed to Step #2.

Step #2 – Decide what's the best option for the individual

Whoever the person is, the decision to have a sex change or not should benefit him/her. All aspects must be considered when arriving at a final decision. Don't just deal with the present, try to foresee what will happen in the future. Would your decision be beneficial to the person in the long run? If you're the person concerned, would it be good for you?

Step #3 – Undergo psychotherapy

Whether you've decided for you or the person concerned to have a sex change or to stick to the assigned gender, you have to prepare your mind and undergo psychotherapy. The purpose is to allow you to inculcate in your mind the reality of what your gender is.

If you have decided to stick to the assigned gender, you have to undergo several sessions of psychotherapy to change your mind set. In this

20

instance, it will be difficult since the cause is perceived to be biological, and the effective treatment is expected to be biological in nature as well. This also applies to other persons.

In instances when sex change is the person's decision, psychotherapy is good in ensuring that the transition to the other gender goes smoothly.

Step #4 - Start hormone therapy

You can start the hormone therapy whether the person has decided to recognize his/her assigned gender or have a sex change. When the person has decided to stay with his or her assigned gender, taking hormones will strengthen and develop the secondary sexual characteristics.

On the other hand, if the decision is a female-to-male sex change, male hormones are given to the person to prepare her for the transformation and the surgical procedure. The same runs true with the male-to-female sex change; female hormones are given to prepare the body for a female transformation and enhance female secondary sexual characteristics.

If you're the person with Gender Dysphoria, all of these will apply to you.

Step #5 – Live as the other gender for at least 1 year

This is required to determine whether the selected gender does indeed fit the person's way of living and character. This is the social gender role transition, which is a crucial step that has to be taken regardless of whether the person has decided to stay with his assigned gender or undergo a sex change. However, the continual psychotherapy and counseling given at this time should be in line with the gender the person has chosen.

Step #6 – Sex-change surgery is performed

After Step #5, the specialist performs the sex-change surgery that the person has selected. The person then becomes the desired gender and will be commonly known as a transgender.

Before the surgery the person must not only be prepared physically but mentally too, and should be oriented positively with regard to the following concepts:

- A person with gender dysphoria is not mentally retarded or deranged. Often, people with Gender Dysphoria are mistakenly regarded as psychiatrically-ill patients. Even though, there are instances in which some persons with Gender Dysphoria also have a mental illness. Gender Dysphoria per se is NOT a mental disorder (illness).

- The person's feeling of anxiety, distress and depression are genuine. He's not imagining it, there's a scientific basis for these emotions.

23

Hence, they must not be disregarded or ignored.

- What gender the individual becomes in the end is not the entire persona. Whatever the gender is, the true worth of a person lies in their personality and character. This must be emphasized to the person with Gender Dysphoria. It is character that counts most!

- The person must maintain an optimistic attitude. This is because being positive about things will help him/her experience the transformation as a happier and smoother process. The people around him should also be positive about the process.

For more information about the sex change process, you may consider also reading one of the following books, also available on Amazon:

- *Sex Change – Male to Female*

  Here's the link to download: www.amazon.com/dp/B013GKON4O/

- *Sex Change – Female to Male*

  Here's the link to download: www.amazon.com/dp/B013GKOQEG/

In instances where surgery is not chosen, a continual hormonal therapy (recommended by a health specialist) can be given based on the person's final gender choice.

Step #7 – Enlist support of family and friends

After the sex-change surgery, the support of the person's family and friends is of significant assistance to the person's return to a normal life. His/her choice must be respected and supported. If the person has no ability to decide for himself or herself, like in the case of children or minors, the guardian must decide for him/her.

Step #8 – Sign up with a support group

Signing up with a support group can allow the person to learn from the experiences of people who are dealing with the same condition. Members can understand and help one other.

Step #9 – Monitor developments

The progress of the person must be monitored and documented. This will allow corrective measures, such as hormonal treatment, psychotherapy or counseling to be instituted whenever the need arises. Monitoring will help the person maintain the gender selected, and move on with their life.

These are the steps that a person can follow when coping with Gender Dysphoria. The steps should serve as guides in dealing with the condition.

Chapter 3: Home Management Strategies

Family members at home can assist enormously in the management of persons with Gender Dysphoria. All members must be informed of the condition and learn how to deal with it. Here's a list of the strategies you can do at home.

1. **Express your support through your actions**

   Let the person know that you're not ashamed of his/her decision. This is one way of expressing your support. Don't apologize to people for your family member's Gender Dysphoria. You must also show respect to the person who has Gender Dysphoria.

2. **Provide family time**

   You should spend time with family members to support the member with Gender

Dysphoria. Family members have to shower the person with unconditional love no matter what decision he has arrived at. This family time will be an actual demonstration of the family's love and concern for the member with the condition.

3. Provide a healthy atmosphere

The ambiance at home has to be normal and healthy with no degrading remarks or snide comments about the person's gender choice. After all, a good person is not based on one's gender.

4. Let the person feel that he truly belongs

Family members must demonstrate love and concern for the persons with Gender Dysphoria so that they can truly feel a sense of belonging. There must be no discrimination, and the preferred gender must be acknowledged and addressed appropriately.

5. Help the person socialize

Helping the person socialize with friends and the society as a whole is one task family members must not ignore. If family members show people their love and concern for the person, despite his/her condition, people will also treat the person in a similar manner.

6. Give unconditional love

The person needs your unconditional love more than anything else. This means that there are no conditions set to gain love. Let the person know that whatever the ultimate decision is; whichever gender the person is, there will always be love.

These are the steps you can take at home to help the Gender Dysphoric person. You must consider these as necessary steps in dealing with the person.

Chapter 4: Medical Intervention Options

There are three most common medical interventions applied to persons with Gender Dysphoria; these are psychotherapy, hormonal therapy and surgical procedures. Below are the details of these methods.

Psychotherapy

Even though Gender Dysphoria is now not considered a mental disorder, psychotherapy is still needed for the psychological adjustment of the person in coping with his/her condition. Take note that the psychotherapist must be duly accredited. You can enlist the help of the yellow pages or persons who have undergone treatment to recommend a competent psychotherapist who's familiar with transgender individuals. In addition, it's preferable that he has had training in counseling, since the sessions will consist of verbal exchanges between the person and the therapist. This will help channel useful and positive thoughts towards the gender selected by the individual.

Psychotherapists often combine two or more methods, such as Cognitive Behavioral Therapy (CBT), behavior modification and systematic desensitization to help people overcome their Gender Dysphoria.

Cognitive Behavioral Therapy

In CBT, the thought patterns and behavior of the person concerned is altered to coincide with the desired behavioral outcomes. So, in Gender Dysphoria, the person will be introduced to ideas, thoughts and behavior that are expected from the specific gender chosen by the individual.

Behavior Modification

Behavior modification is similar to CBT but focuses on the cultivation of the positive behavior expected from the person.

Systematic Desensitization

On the other hand, systematic desensitization is the exposure of the person to the stimulus that he fears until he gets used to it. This can be utilized when the person has decided to stay with his/her assigned gender instead of undergoing sex-change surgery.

Hormonal Therapy

The development of secondary sexual characteristics of each individual depends upon his/her sexual hormones. This is more effective if undergone before puberty. The female gonadal hormones namely, estrogen and progesterone are typically given to persons who want to enhance or develop female traits, while the male gonadal hormones namely, testosterone and androgens are given to persons who would like to develop and enhance their male characteristics.

The concentration of the hormone given will depend on the recommendation of the doctor. The dosage can depend on the age and weight of the individual as well as the gravity of the Gender Dysphoria. The dosage for testosterone (testosterone cypionate) is 200 milligrams administered intramuscularly (IM) every 2 weeks. The dosage for estrogen (conjugated estrogen) is 7.5 to 10 milligrams per deciliter administered intramuscularly or orally every 2 weeks or as prescribed by the medical doctor. However, you should be aware of the side effects of hormonal therapy.

Side effects of hormonal therapy:

- Increased risk of the formation of gall stones
- Sleep apnea or interrupted breathing during sleep
- Potential formation of blood clots, which can be life-threatening
- Propensity towards obesity
- Formation of acne on skin
- Danger of becoming infertile

Surgical procedures

There are several surgical procedures that can be performed, if the person finally undergoes sex-change surgeries. Here are some of the most common surgical procedures. Again, for more information about these procedures and their impacts, please refer to the **'Sex Change – Male to Female'** and **'Sex Change – Female to Male'** books recommended in the previous chapter.

Sex Change – Male to Female:
http://www.amazon.com/dp/B013GKON4O/

Sex Change – Female to Male:
http://www.amazon.com/dp/B013GKOQEG/

Male-to-female sex change

1. **Penectomy** – To make way for the construction of the vagina, the penis is surgically removed or excised.

2. **Orchidectomy** – A uterus will take the place of the testes, which is surgically removed to make the male more feminine.

3. **Breast implantation** – The breasts are major physical features that females possess; hence, artificial breasts are surgically implanted in the man's chest area. These implants are commonly made of a special synthetic or silicon material.

4. **Clitoroplasty** – The clitoris is labeled as the center of erotic pleasures in the female body and without it, a person cannot be a genuine female. So, as a trans-female, the surgical construction of the clitoris is essential.

5. **Vulvoplasty** – The vulva is a vital part of the female anatomy. The creation of the vulva has to be included in the surgical construction of the female sexual organs.

6. **Vaginoplasty** – This is where the penis penetrates during sexual intercourse, and without it, a trans-female cannot call herself a true female. Vaginal construction has to be a part of the procedure.

38

7. **Facial reconstruction** – With the surgical reconstruction of the facial features, the person will look more feminine, and the transformation will be complete.

Female-to-male sex change

1. **Hysterectomy** – The uterus makes women distinctive from men because of it is childbearing organ. With the surgical removal of the uterus, the trans-male can truly feel like a man.

2. **Mastectomy** – The breasts are important to women but not to men. It's a feminine physical trait that trans-males must get rid of through surgical removal.

3. **Scrotoplasty** – Males without balls aren't masculine. Hence, through the surgical construction of the scrotum, the trans-male will feel and see that he's indeed a man.

4. **Phalloplasty** - The phallus (penis) is the ultimate male organ. Some people measure

manhood by the presence of a penis. This process involves the surgical construction of the penis from tissues taken from the inner forearm, vagina or lower abdomen. The clitoris can also be enhanced through hormonal therapy to become a penis.

5. **Salpingo-oophorectomy** – This process involves the surgical removal of the ovaries and the fallopian tubes, which are important parts of the female reproductive system. The ovaries produce eggs or ova for fertilization by the male. With their removal, the childbearing characteristic of women will no longer exist.

6. **Facial reconstruction** – Through surgery, female facial features are eliminated and made more masculine. This operation will be up to the decision of the person.

These are the medical interventions that persons with Gender Dysphoria can opt to undergo. Surgical procedures may have physical AND mental side effects. Hence, the person must prepare himself or herself physically and mentally to undergo the procedure.

Chapter 5: Laws Protecting Transgender Rights

There are laws that protect transsexual persons or transgenders against abuse and discrimination. You must be aware of them, so you or the person with Gender Dysphoria can avoid unnecessary abuse.

1. Equality Act 2010

If the persons with Gender Dysphoria are living in the UK, they can invoke this act to protect their rights. This act includes the rights of transsexuals in their working environment and in society against discrimination, victimization and harassment. The laws found in the Sexual Discrimination Act 1975 are included in this act.

2. Gender Recognition Act 2004

This act will recognize the person's gender legally. They just have to apply for a new gender identity certificate. Persons can also apply for a new birth certificate, passport and driver's license. However, they must be 18 years of age or above, and must prove that they have Gender Dysphoria, and have undergone sex change. They must also prove that they have lived as a transsexual for 2 years or more. Consequently, they must demonstrate that they will live that way for the rest of their lives.

3. World Professional Association for Transgender Health (WPATH) Guidelines in Treating Transsexuals

These guidelines are designed for health professionals, who are tapped in treating transsexuals. These guidelines protect the rights of transsexuals and ensure fair and competent treatment when undergoing medical consultations and procedures.

4. Equal Opportunity in Education Act

This act was created in America in 2014 to protect the rights of transgenders or transsexuals. But officially only 13 states and the District of Columbia have implemented non-discrimination laws, which are explicit for transsexuals. These states are New Jersey, Iowa, Massachusetts, California, Washington, Minnesota, Vermont, Colorado, New York, Illinois, Connecticut, Oregon and Maine.

Nevada, New Mexico, Maryland, Hawaii, Delaware, and Rhode Island have laws against the discrimination of transgenders but they differ on the coverage. Likewise with Michigan, New York, Indiana, Pennsylvania and Kentucky; they have laws against the discrimination of state workers who are transgenders.

The other states have laws that protect transgenders against discrimination but these are not explicitly stated and categorized because of opposition from certain groups. You will have to get in touch with the local government in your state to know more about the person's rights as a transgender in your area.

5. Civil Rights Act

Although this law wasn't created specifically for transsexuals, it's a law that you can cite to ward off discrimination. This act includes the prohibition of discrimination based on gender, and this encompasses your rights as a transgender.

These are all the laws that can protect a person who has Gender Dysphoria when applying for work, having a medical check-up or when performing other vital activities. Federals laws regarding people with gender Dysphoria vary from state to state, so make sure you know the specific laws affecting your specific state.

Chapter 6:   Important Pointers to Keep in Mind

The resolution of the problem caused by Gender Dysphoria will depend a lot on the person having the condition. Here are some essential pointers that you can quickly refer to, when in doubt.

1. **The person with Gender Dysphoria must first try psychotherapy and hormonal treatment.** Deciding to undergo sex change without undergoing psychotherapy and hormonal treatment that is in line with the assigned gender is reckless. Take note that there are instances where persons have remained with their assigned gender after hormonal therapy and psychotherapy.

2. **Psychotherapy is crucial before and after sex change.** The mind is a powerful tool that can help you succeed or fail in any endeavor, so don't disregard it. The person has to be psychologically prepared for any procedure to succeed.

3. **The person must create a strong support group.** This is crucial for a transgender to succeed. The support group can be composed of family members, trusted friends, a competent counselor or psychotherapist, and a group of people with the same condition. Connection with this support group should be continuous.

4. **One of the most difficult stages is the adjustment to society once sex change happens.** This phase involves all aspects of a person's life: their career, social life and family. Individuals will need all the support they can obtain after the sex change surgery.

5. **The person must have a positive frame of mind.** When resolving Gender Dysphoria, the person has to be optimistic because there will be various setbacks encountered. The positive behavior will help him stay determined and patient in achieving his goal.

6. **There can be periods of remission in the process.** This means that a person with Gender Dysphoria may accept his/her assigned gender or birth gender. In this phase, the guardian can use hormonal therapy to

strengthen the assigned gender to avoid sex change. Even though the strategy doesn't have a high probability of success, it may be effective in children.

7. **Avoid derogatory statements about the person's Gender Dysphoria.** Cruel words are more painful than physical wounds because they last forever. This is especially true with children and teenagers, whom are more susceptible.

8. **Dealing with Gender Dysphoria at an early age can resolve the problem quicker.** If you notice symptoms in a child, ensure that you institute steps to resolve it at the onset. You can consult a team of health specialists to help you deal with the condition.

9. **Undiagnosed Gender Dysphoria can lead to illnesses**. If the condition is not diagnosed accurately and treated accordingly, anxiety and depression can occur. This may later on lead to more serious conditions, such as schizophrenia and serious mental depression.

10. **Hormonal intake must only be done through a doctor's recommendation.** Hormones have profound effects on the body's biological functions, so they should not be ingested without a prescription. Even a small amount of these potent substances can affect the body significantly.

11. **After a sex change surgery, the person has to continue his/her counseling.** This is to ensure that his/her transformation is complete and is continuous.

12. **Exercise can increase the male hormone, testosterone.** If the person is a trans-male, he can exercise daily to increase his testosterone levels. This is a risk-free method of becoming more masculine.

13. **Be aware that there are rights for people with Gender Dysphoria.** The persons must know what they are entitled to, so that discrimination will not occur. Kindly refer to Chapter 5.

14. **Deciding whether to live with the birth gender or to be a transgender is a**

momentous decision. The decision must be made over several years of careful self-evaluation and retrospection.

15. **Gender Dysphoria is now universally-known.** Despite people's awareness of the condition, there are some people who are still opposed to sex change. But the good news is that the percentage of acceptance is increasing.

Combine these recommendations along with the other information provided in this book and you can triumph over your battle in dealing with this condition.

Conclusion

Gender Dysphoria can be resolved by two ways; the individuals can choose to stay with their birth or assigned gender, or they can undergo a sex change. This will depend on the persons concerned, or the guardians, in cases of minors. It's important that the concerned persons' feelings are considered because the decision will affect their lives for as long as they live.

Following the recommendations in this book can help you deal with Gender Dysphoria, if you implement them correctly. You can also modify them to suit the individual's personality. These recommendations are not written in stone, but they should be followed wisely and responsibly.

Remember, if the decision is to stay with the birth gender, children and teens before the age of puberty have better chances of treatment, while adults commonly succeed with sex changes.

If sex change is the answer to the predicament, continue with the procedure with enough confidence. The success rate is pegged at 97%, so, generally there's a minimal 3% rate of failure. The failure is caused by not continuing with counseling, psychotherapy and the prescribed cross-hormonal treatment.

Hence, don't allow Gender Dysphoria to affect you negatively. There are now effective ways to resolve the issue. Hopefully, you can deal successfully with yours, or your family member's Gender Dysphoria.

Finally, I'd like to thank you for purchasing this book! If you found it helpful, I'd greatly appreciate it if you'd take a moment to leave a review on Amazon. Thank you!